# PERIOD POWER
## Fact about menstrual cycle and its principle

Jennifer perry

# Table of content

# Chapter 1

The bloody truth and what you need to know

The menstrual cycle: what is it?

Your body prepares for pregnancy by going through the menstrual cycle. This cycle spans the day before the beginning of your subsequent menstruation to the first day of your period (the first day of bleeding).

Typically, ovulation occurs in the second part of the cycle. When one of your ovaries releases an egg, this occurs. The egg must be fertilized by the sperm to become pregnant.

Not every woman experiences ovulation every month. Some disorders, such as endometriosis and polycystic ovarian syndrome, may prevent ovulation from occurring (PCOS). Consult your doctor if you are attempting to become pregnant but not having a monthly period.

How long does a cycle of menses last?

Although the typical duration of a woman's cycle is around 28 days, it may vary from month to month and in length. Regular cycles that are either longer or shorter than this are common (from 21 to 41 days).

No matter how long your cycle is, the majority of women ovulate between 10 and 16 days before the beginning of their subsequent menstrual period.

When in my cycle may I get pregnant?

It is possible, although unusual, to get pregnant just before or right after your period. When you ovulate, when you are most fertile, is also the time when you are most likely to get pregnant. You may find the optimum days to become pregnant by understanding your cycle and learning more about what happens each month.

Learn more about ovulation and fertility, as well as the best advice for identifying your fertile window. To learn more, you may also use our ovulation calculator.

What happens if my cycle is erratic?

Because you may not ovulate consistently if you have irregular periods, becoming pregnant may be more challenging.

Your fertility may be impacted by irregular periods, which have a wide range of potential reasons. For instance:

• Significant weight gain or decrease

• anxiety or excessive exercise

• medical diseases such as polycystic ovary syndrome or thyroid issues.

Even though you may have irregular periods, there are steps you may do to increase your chances of becoming pregnant.

Consult your doctor if you're having trouble conceiving and your periods have stopped, are irregular, or you're missing your monthly cycle.

I have been using birth control. My cycle will be impacted by this.

How you've been utilizing contraception will determine this. Try to allow yourself up to three months for your natural menstrual cycle to return to its "normal rhythm" if you've been using the pill since your period may be erratic when you first stop taking it.

A "withdrawal bleed" is the first menstruation that comes after discontinuing the medication. Your first natural menstruation comes following this.

The injection of birth control may potentially alter your monthly cycle. Your menstrual cycle might alter, becoming heavier, shorter, lighter, or stopping entirely. Even after you stop getting injections, this may persist for a few months.

Your fertility will return to normal if you utilize the contraceptive implant as soon as it is removed.

How soon after stopping the pill may I get pregnant?

You can get pregnant as soon as you stop taking the pill, but it's a good idea to wait until you've had a regular period if you're trying to conceive. This will allow your body time to adapt and an opportunity for you to determine if you're prepared for pregnancy. Check out your options with our pregnancy planning tool.

My menstrual cycle continues to be erratic. My fertility has been impacted by the pill.

Although it's doubtful that the pill has affected fertility, it may sometimes mask

issues you already experience, including irregular periods or PCOS.

This is because, although it's common to have period-like bleeding when taking the pill, you don't have a period. Instead, the tablet inhibits the ovaries from producing an egg (ovulation).

If your periods are still irregular 3 months after ceasing contraception, see your doctor.

Can I determine my due date using my menstrual cycle?

Yes. By counting backward from the first day of your most recent period, you may determine how far along you are in your pregnancy (and, therefore, when the baby is due).

This might be perplexing as you most likely didn't get pregnant until around two weeks after you ovulated. Even if you are aware of the exact day you become pregnant, if your cycle is 28 days long, this counts as day 14 rather than day 1 of your pregnancy.

Because your body prepares for pregnancy each time you have a period, your pregnancy is determined by the date of your most recent menstrual cycle. It also provides a benchmark for medical practitioners to adhere to since it may be exceedingly difficult to pinpoint the precise moment the sperm fertilized the egg.

It will be more difficult to determine your due date if your cycle is erratic or if you've just started taking the pill.

When you are between 11 and 14 weeks pregnant, an ultrasound is the best approach to determine your due date. This is done to assess your growth and that of your unborn child.

Despite being pregnant, I am bleeding. If so, when am I due?

When a woman is pregnant, implantation bleeding may sometimes occur around the time her period should have arrived. During implantation, the growing embryo embeds itself in the uterine wall. A very faint bleeding (spotting) called an implantation bleed is often pinkish and sometimes brown. Everybody won't have an implantation bleed.

Before 12 weeks, it's normal to have minor bleeding or "spotting" without any discomfort. Even while this isn't usually dangerous, you should still be checked out right away by your doctor, midwife, or early pregnancy unit.

# Chapter 2

What may go wrong with your periods and period poverty

It is a worldwide problem that affects everyone.
All around the globe, menstruating people are excluded from simple activities like socializing and eating certain foods. Women are discouraged from attending school and working every day because of the social stigma associated with menstruation and a lack of resources. Lack of access to sanitary products, education on menstrual hygiene, latrines, handwashing stations, or waste disposal is referred to as period poverty.

Period products are now considered to be as necessary as toilet paper in several nations, states, and localities throughout the globe. However, more has to be done. Menstrual products were just made free in US federal prisons in 2018. In addition, a 2017 survey revealed that almost 1 in 5 females had skipped class because they couldn't get period supplies.

However, initiatives to acknowledge period poverty as a pressing problem have advanced. The world's top professionals in the field will gather to define objectives for menstruation advocacy at the first global conference on period poverty, which is scheduled to begin in Australia in October 2022.

"A major problem of human rights, dignity, and public health is meeting the hygienic requirements of all teenage females.

Poor menstruation hygiene is not only a concern for women in the US. Both wealthy and developing countries are affected, and poor women are more susceptible.

Here is all the information you want on this grave human rights issue.

The 3 Most Important Facts About Period Poverty

• Reproductive and urinary tract infections have been related to poor menstrual hygiene, which may have negative effects on physical health.

• 1.7 billion people worldwide lack access to basic sanitary services.

• A disproportionate number of girls with disabilities lack access to the facilities and materials required for good menstrual hygiene.

People Affected

Menstrual health is a problem that affects both sexes. 1.7 billion people worldwide lack access to basic sanitary services. Nearly 75 percent of individuals in underdeveloped nations lack access to even the most basic handwashing facilities at home. It is more difficult for women and young girls to manage their periods safely and respectably when they are unable to utilize these facilities.

More often than not, girls with disabilities lack access to the facilities and supplies necessary for good menstrual hygiene. Women and girls may find it more challenging to control their periods while living in war zones or in communities that have recently experienced a natural catastrophe.

Even young males might benefit from learning about menstruation hygiene. Early menstrual education in the home and at school encourages healthy behaviors and removes stigmas associated with the normal process. To achieve menstruation equality, everyone must have access to sanitary products, suitable restrooms, hand-washing stations, sanitation and hygiene education, and waste management.

What Causes Predominate?

The menstrual cycle is stigmatized everywhere. Some societies consider menstruation women to be unclean and confine them to huts while they are menstruating. Menstrual huts are legally against the law, but because of deeply ingrained cultural assumptions, families continue to take the chance.

According to research by the non-governmental organization WoMena, many females skip class when they are on their period to avoid being teased by their peers.

Many women and adolescents also struggle to pay for menstruation supplies. The widespread promotion of the color pink to women is the origin of the term "pink tax," which refers to the tampon fee. While some nations have eliminated the tax on period products as luxury goods, others still utilize it as a means of gender discrimination. However, eliminating the tax globally won't make period products accessible on their own since too many people can't afford them and often have to choose between buying food or menstruation supplies.

According to the United Nations International Children's Emergency Fund, many families in Bangladesh cannot afford menstruation supplies and instead use old clothes (UNICEF). According to the Indian Ministry of Health, just 12% of menstruators in India have access to sanitary items, forcing the other 82% to utilize harmful substitutes like rags and sawdust.

Why Does It Matter?

According to UNICEF, poor menstrual hygiene has been connected to reproductive and urinary tract infections as well as physical health hazards. Women are also prevented from achieving their full potential when they pass up chances that are essential to their development. Lack of education among young girls increases their likelihood of underage marriages, early pregnancy, malnutrition, domestic abuse, and pregnancy difficulties.

Shame over periods also has detrimental mental impacts. It weakens women by making them feel ashamed of a typical biological function.

How can we prevent it?

Menstruation must be normalized to break taboos associated with the regular process. Then, legislation must be put into effect to ensure that hygiene, sanitation, and menstruation products are freely available.

Menstrual equality policy is being prioritized by activists and supporters, although traditionally, it has been difficult to address.

# Chapter 3

Taking care of oneself

Cramps, bloating, exhaustion, and other unpleasant symptoms are more prevalent at this time of the month. throughout the week of your period to acknowledge, enjoy, and reconnect with your body.

1. Provide your body with meals high in iron.

Cycle-syncing, or altering your lifestyle following your monthly hormonal swings, is probably a concept you've heard of. In other words, The Cycle Syncing Method® advises varying your routine to meet your body's demands as they relate to the various periods of your menstrual cycle.

Your hormone levels decrease throughout the menstrual phase, often known as your period, leaving you feeling lethargic. Fill your plate with meals high in iron and nutrients, and make sure you're getting enough calories. Consider wild salmon, steak, chicken, or turkey as possible sources of protein. Vegetarian or vegan? No issue! Stock up on pinto beans, chickpeas, and lentils. Of course, we must not neglect vegetables. This week, think of kale, spinach, and other dark, leafy greens as your greatest pals. Finally, for an extra blast of anti-inflammatory goodness, add herbs and spices like cinnamon, ginger, and turmeric to your foods.

Keep hydrated.
Hydration is important, particularly at this period, so you know now is the time to get that inspirational water bottle you've been talking about. Replace your cup of coffee with a non-caffeinated tea, such as red raspberry leaf tea, to give your coffee maker a rest. The red raspberry leaf is a rich source of calcium, iron, potassium, and vitamins A, C, and E. Not quite persuaded? According to research, red raspberry leaves may lessen

the pelvic muscular spasms that produce menstruation cramps.

3. Be cautious while working out.

Have you ever noticed how alluring your bed gets when your period starts? Even while staying in bed all week isn't practical, pay attention to your body and steer clear of any intense activities. Put a stop to any Rocky-inspired exercises, marathon training, or HIIT regimens. Instead, choose softer, low-impact exercises like stretching, Pilates, restorative yoga, or walking. Or go for a leisurely trek, jog, or swim outside to release endorphins while absorbing vitamin D. being active during your period indeed has numerous advantages, such as reducing tiredness and mood swings, but if you're very exhausted, having a rest day or two is perfectly acceptable.

4. Schedule relaxation time on your schedule.

It might be challenging—even uncomfortable—to permit yourself to relax when you're used to a fast-paced, go-go-go existence. Even if you may be used to working a 60-hour work week or double-booking your schedule, this week is not the time to push yourself to the limit. Instead, use this week to take it easy and give yourself some me time. Reduce the number of work meetings and social engagements on your calendar, schedule time for a warm bath or massage, indulge in some sex if you're up for it, or romance yourself with some self-love if it's not in the cards, ground yourself by going outside, and maximize your sleep by keeping your bedroom cool and restraining that urge.

5. Let rid of everything that could be preventing you.

It's time to focus on yourself and let go of anything that is no longer helping you, whether it be people, habits, beliefs, or a career, much as the uterus loses its lining during the week before your period. Your level of clarity and intuition are at their highest during this period, making it the best time to reflect on your life and digest your decisions. What things that prevent you from becoming your best self can you let go of? And what room can you make by doing this? To help you live your greatest life, try including writing, manifestation, or meditation.

6. Take into account substitute menstruation products

Today, there are many creative and environmentally friendly alternatives to conventional period items, making the move simpler than ever. Before your period starts again, think about using menstrual cups, menstrual discs, or period underwear as alternatives to traditional feminine care products.

# Chapter 4

Period relief

Can Home Remedies Treat Menstrual Cramps?

Most of the time, women may cure period cramps at home.

Don't be scared to speak with your doctor if your pain is significant and interfering with your daily activities. You may need more therapy or prescription-only medications to become well.

These natural home treatments for menstrual cramp relief are safe and efficient in easing period discomfort.

1. Practice Yoga Pose to Reduce Period Pain

Regular yoga practice may alleviate cramps, whether it's due to the soothing effects of the postures or the stretching of your muscles.

You may practice between periods or while you're having one, although some teachers caution against avoiding inverted positions (m 2. Curl Up With a Heating Pad to Ease Period Cramps

"Since the uterus is a muscle, anything that aids in muscular relaxation, such as administering heat, might be helpful."
Studies indicated that topical ibuprofen for period pains was effective, as reported in Evidence-Based Nursing. The ladies were given heat alone, heat + ibuprofen, ibuprofen alone, or a placebo during the two research days. The group that received both heat and ibuprofen had the greatest outcomes; adding heat accelerated recovery.

3. Take a secure pain reliever to reduce inflammation.

One of the best strategies to manage period pain is to moderately take nonsteroidal anti-inflammatory (NSAID) drugs like ibuprofen (Advil, Motrin), or naproxen (Aleve). NSAIDs do this by lowering prostaglandin levels in the body. Because of this, taking medication just before your period might prevent the amount of pain-causing prostaglandins from increasing.

As with any medication, you should first speak to your doctor to ensure if NSAIDs are a suitable fit for you, particularly if you have a history of bleeding or stomach, renal, or other health concerns.

Your doctor may advise you to take an NSAID with more power if the over-the-counter NSAIDs you purchase are insufficiently relieving. For cramps, some women need up to 800 milligrams three times each day. To do that, you would need to take a lot of over-the-counter medications.

## 4. Some types of herbal tea may ease cramping

Some drinks might ease menstruation cramps

Despite the paucity of research on the topic, menstruation women have long utilized tea as a pain reliever in many cultures.

## 5. Increase Your Magnesium Intake

The discomfort of cramps seems to be lessened by dietary magnesium.
Numerous foods, such as almonds, black beans, spinach, yogurt, and peanut butter, contain magnesium.

Meet with your doctor if you wish to take a magnesium supplement since the dosage you need depends on the frequency and intensity of your cramps, among other things.

## 6. Essential Oil Massage for Pain Relief

Menstrual cramps may be eased by massaging your skin with particular fragrant essential oils.
Be careful to use essential oils carefully. Purchase tested-purity oils of superior quality.

## 7. Exercise Will Increase Your Feel-Good Endorphins (or Orgasm)

Natural endorphins produced by the body are believed to improve mood. They also have a pain-killing effect, however. Aerobic exercise is a common strategy to increase endorphin production. An orgasm is still another.

8. Birth control medications may also lessen uncomfortable cramping

Birth control pills and hormonal intrauterine devices, although not precisely a home treatment, are possible tools in your anti cramping toolbox and should not be disregarded.

Consider the reduction of cramps as a benefit of several forms of contraception. When they start taking the pill, many women get relief from excruciating cramps. Hormonal birth control often reduces bleeding, and reduced bleeding might result in fewer cramps.